ALL ABOUT POISONOUS PLANTS

CONTENTS

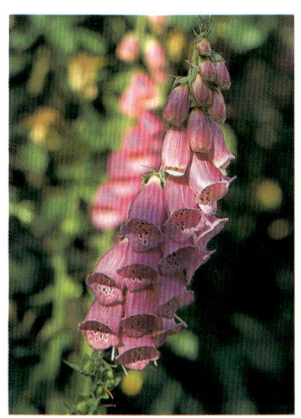

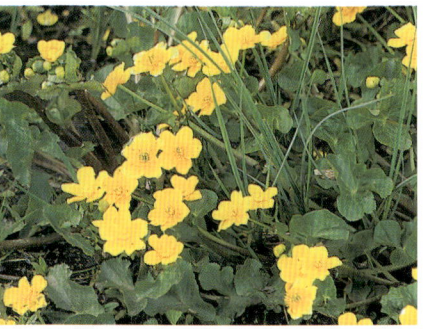

W0082673

Disclaimer

There is still controversy over which plants are a risk to horses, and there are hundreds of potentially dangerous plants I have been unable to include in this book which is a guide to those plants most commonly encountered. If you are in any doubt about the identification of poisonous plants, consult a botanist and take veterinary advice. Always wear gloves when handling poisonous plants and keep them away from eyes and faces.

INTRODUCTION

Horses are particularly vulnerable to poisoning from plants as their diet is solely vegetable matter. If harmful food is eaten, the toxins ingested must pass through the body as a horse is unable to vomit. In the wild, horses can roam for miles and have access to the food of their choice, so the often bitter-tasting dangerous plants are usually ignored. Semi-domesticated animals such as horses depend on their owners to provide the correct diet as restricted grazing prevents them choosing for themselves.

WHY HORSES EAT POISONOUS PLANTS

There are many circumstances in which horses may choose to eat, or be unable to avoid eating, unsuitable plants.

When they are hungry
• From starvation resulting from severe food shortage • From imposed diets for overweight animals • When an expected feed arrives a few hours later than normal.

When they are tired of dry food
• After a long winter • Following a hot summer which has burnt the grass • After months on a very high concentrate diet.

If the plants are palatable
• When young, some toxic plants are not so bitter and, if in the spring they grow more quickly than grass, then they will be tempting • Other plants lose their bitter taste but not their toxicity when processed in hay or dried at the end of the summer • Herbicides can make some plants more palatable for a few weeks, therefore chemically treated land should be rested for a while.

Through human ignorance
• 'Helpful' neighbours may tip poisonous hedge clippings and garden refuse into the field.

From the novelty factor – gaining access to new plants
• Deadly roots can be exposed during drainage work • Snow can weigh down poisonous branches so they are in reach • A tethered horse may eat everything within reach including poisonous bark • Horses moved to different fields may experiment with new and dangerous plants • Fallen branches can create a new danger.

As a result of addiction
• Horses can become addicted to poisonous plants (e.g. ragwort, foxglove, oak, acorns and bracken) in the same way that humans become addicted to alcohol or drugs.

From overexposure to one plant
• It is important that horses have a balanced diet to avoid overconsumption of plants which would be beneficial rather than toxic if consumed in small quantities.

HIDDEN IN HAY

Plants to watch out for in hay include ragwort, bracken, cowbane, foxglove, horsetails, iris, lupins and meadow saffron.

SUSPECTED POISONING

Symptoms of poisoning often involve colic, convulsions, lack of co-ordination and changes in temperature, pulse and respiration. If plant poisoning is ever suspected, seek veterinary advice immediately and, if possible, collect a sample of the plant. Remove animals from the potential source of poisoning. Do not attempt diagnosis or treatment yourself.

RISK OF POISONING

Every book listing plants poisonous to horses mentions different plants and there is continual debate over which plants pose a threat. This is partly because horses often die from poisoning without a post mortem being carried out, or because the animal may recover from poisoning before a diagnosis is made. In many cases therefore, the true risk of poisoning cannot be accurately assessed. It is also difficult to establish what quantities of a plant a horse must eat before suffering from poisoning. In practice, toxin levels of plants vary greatly at different times of year and in different areas. This book highlights plants with which no chances should be taken and provides enough information on other plants for owners to assess the risk for themselves.

PLANT DESCRIPTION

All the plant name descriptions in this book are listed thus: Common name – botanical name (family) [other common names] e.g.

BRACKEN – *Pteridium aquilinium (Dennstaedtiaceae)* [brake]

spp. = species

MEDICINAL VALUE

Some toxic plants can be used for medicinal purposes in herbal or homeopathic medicine but only in extreme dilution under the advice of an expert.

PASTURE PLANTS

RAGWORT – *Senecio spp. (Compositae)*
There are several species of ragwort. The distinctive yellow flowers and ragged leaves clearly differentiate ragwort from other pasture plants.

Ragwort – *Senecio jacobaea* **[benweed, St James wort, staggerweed and tansy ragwort]**
This species of ragwort causes most of the problems in Britain and is found in abundance throughout the country. It is usually biennial. It can grow to 150 cm and flowers from June to October.

Marsh ragwort – *Senecio aquaticus*
This plant is biennial and prefers damp areas. It flowers between July and August and is between 30 cm and 100 cm in height. The lower leaves have no divisions and have broadly rounded tips.

Hoary ragwort – *Senecio erucifolius*
This perennial is common on road sides and in waste places in south-east England. The leaves have pointed tips and are covered with grey down. Flowers appear around June to October. The height is usually between 30 cm and 100 cm.

Oxford ragwort – *Senecio squalidus*
This species is usually annual and is found in waste places and railway embankments throughout the country. It is smaller than the other ragworts, growing to around 30 cm, and flowers from April to December.

Groundsel – *Senecio vulgaris*
Like S. *jacobaea* this is common in most areas of the country but it is annual and can overwinter. It flowers throughout the year, reaching up to 40 cm.

Ragwort is poisonous at all stages of growth and when dry or in hay. Galloping horses cut the stems allowing them to dry out and become palatable. It has been estimated that ragwort kills more horses than all other poisonous plants put together. Horses can become addicted to ragwort and poisoning is cumulative.

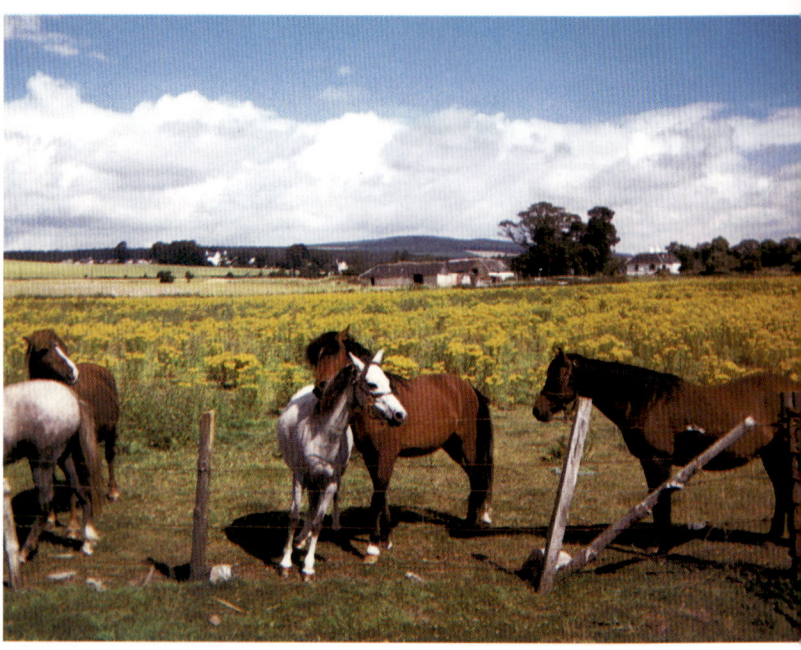

Symptoms of poisoning can appear after one week but are often slow to develop and can even occur when consumption of the plant has ceased. Once clinical signs have appeared death is usually quick. There is no specific treatment as the liver damage is irreversible. Dietary protein, however, should be limited.

HIDDEN LIVER DAMAGE

Low-grade liver damage may only become apparent when the horse's body is under stress, for example when in foal, competing or when ill from other causes.

Local authorities have the power to enforce the 1959 Weeds Act and serve notices requiring a land owner to prevent the plant spreading.

METHODS OF CONTROL

Spraying

Agrochemical suppliers come under the Agricultural Merchants section in *Yellow Pages*, and they will be able to advise on suitable weed killer and equipment. Blanket treatment with herbicide can render pasture unsuitable for grazing for weeks or even months and, as it kills everything, it will leave bare patches where ragwort can easily re-establish itself. However it may be necessary where there is more ragwort than anything else. Recently a revolutionary new plant-based herbicide called Barrier H™ has been licensed. Unlike other herbicides it is effective all year round and, due to its rapid action, horses can be reintroduced to the pasture after as little as two weeks **but, as with other herbicides, only if the foliage has withered and disappeared or any remains are removed**. For most effective use, rosettes should be spot sprayed from September to June. If treating flowering ragwort, a second application may be necessary. Uprooting is probably the method of choice at this stage. For more details see Further Information on page 23.

Uprooting

This is usually done **manually** and is very labour intensive. However, if a few people work together it is surprising how a sea of yellow flowers can quickly be restored to green pasture. Gloves must be worn to allow a good grip and prevent skin irritation. It is important to remove as much of the root as possible: it helps to wiggle the plant from side

The lifecycle shown below is for *S. jacobaea* and indicates the most appropriate method of control for the stage of growth.

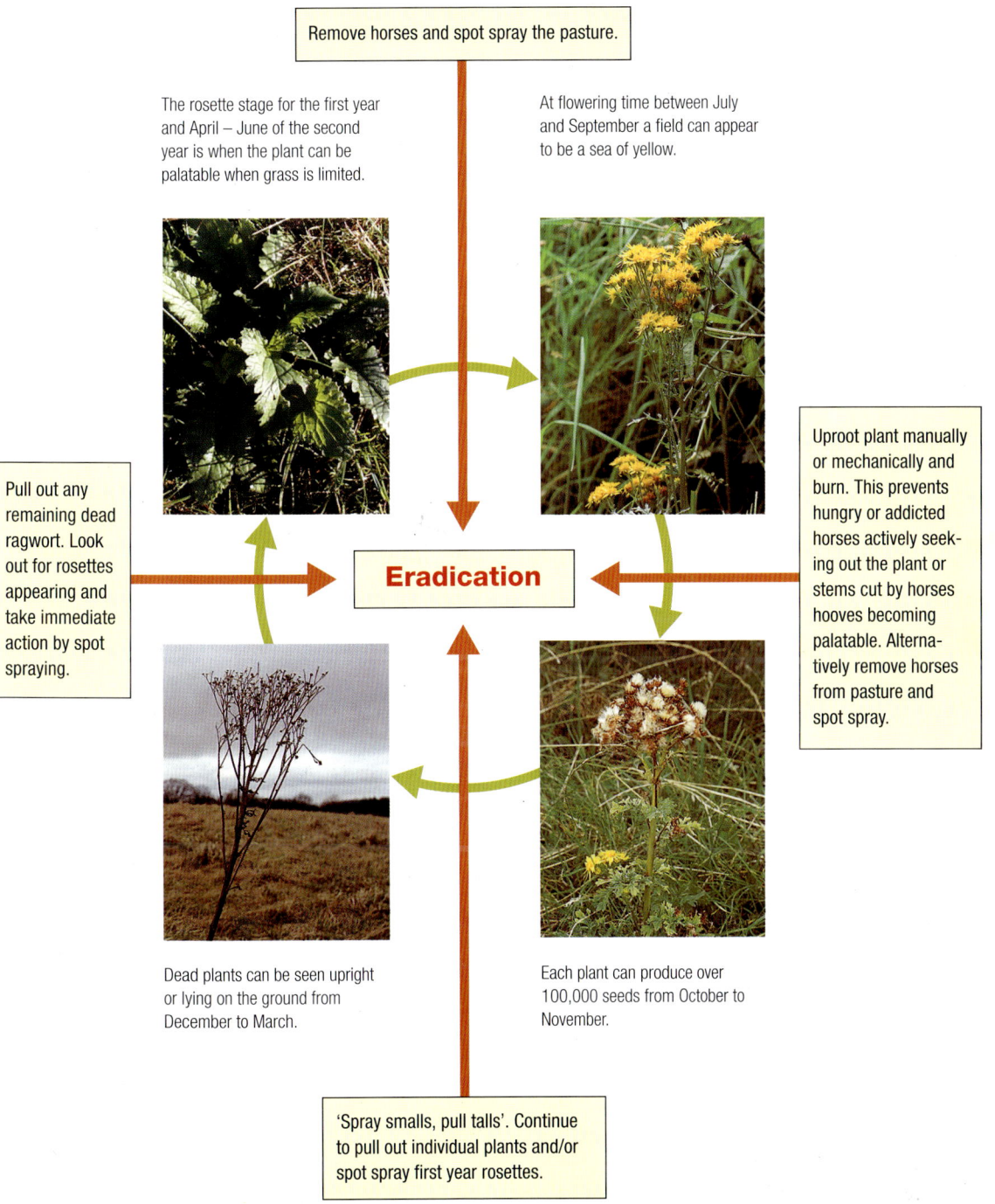

Remove horses and spot spray the pasture.

The rosette stage for the first year and April – June of the second year is when the plant can be palatable when grass is limited.

At flowering time between July and September a field can appear to be a sea of yellow.

Pull out any remaining dead ragwort. Look out for rosettes appearing and take immediate action by spot spraying.

Eradication

Uproot plant manually or mechanically and burn. This prevents hungry or addicted horses actively seeking out the plant or stems cut by horses hooves becoming palatable. Alternatively remove horses from pasture and spot spray.

Dead plants can be seen upright or lying on the ground from December to March.

Each plant can produce over 100,000 seeds from October to November.

'Spray smalls, pull talls'. Continue to pull out individual plants and/or spot spray first year rosettes.

to side before hauling it out. It is ideal to dig out ragwort at the rosette stage although it is difficult to remove all of it at this time. When the first flowers appear the plants are easy to find and it will take a concentrated effort to remove all of them. Then, weekly for the next two months, it will take a short time to pull up the new flowering plants, together with the plants which were previously not properly uprooted and which have re-established. Ragwort can also be uprooted **mechanically**. The Ecopuller manufactured by Alvan Blanch (*see above right*) is a new piece of tractor- or quadbike-towed machinery that can pull out ragwort, thistles and other tall weeds (*see* Acknowledgements).

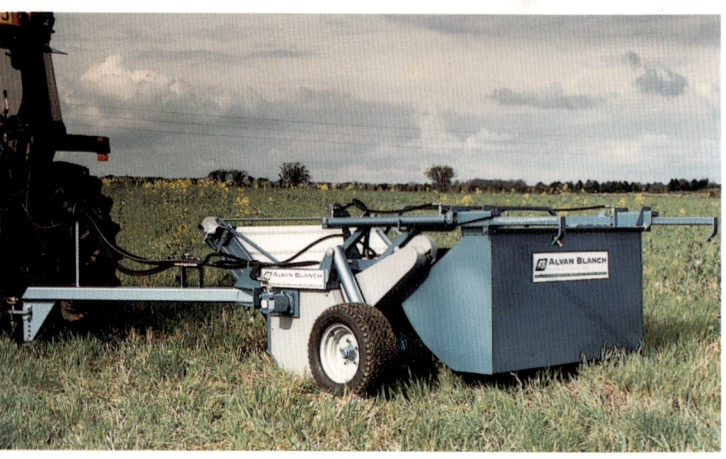

Cutting

Cutting is not effective as the roots of the plant remain in the soil and regrow. It should only be done when the field is not in use to prevent ragwort flowering, seeding and spreading to other land. However, after cutting, the plant will grow even more vigorously the following year. It is vital that all cuttings are lifted to prevent further danger to animals.

Sheep

Ragwort is also toxic to sheep, so some authorities do not consider it acceptable to use sheep to graze rosette-stage ragwort.

Do not take risks with ragwort.

BRACKEN – *Pteridium aquilinum* (*Dennstaedtiaceae*) [brake]

Bracken is a fern with a creeping underground rhizome. It is found in woods and on hills and moors all over the country. The leaves uncurl in the spring (*see below*), grow up to 2 m, and turn brown and die in autumn. If the climate is warm enough, spores are produced from structures on the underside of the leaves in the autumn.

The whole plant is poisonous in all stages of growth and should never be used for bedding or fed in hay. Care must be taken not to

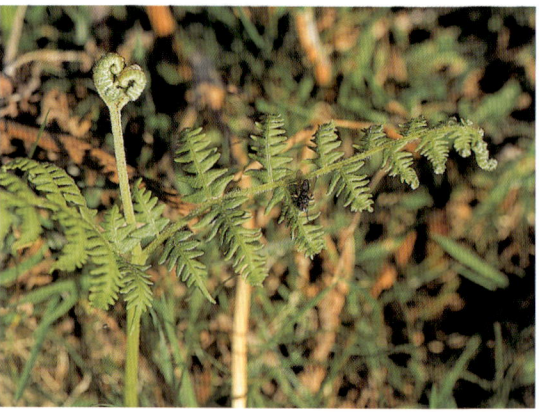

REMOVE AND BURN

Whatever the chosen method of ragwort removal, all plant remnants *must* be removed and burnt.

SPREADING BRACKEN

Bracken continues to spread. Recent estimates suggest that all the bracken in Britain would cover an area the size of Yorkshire.

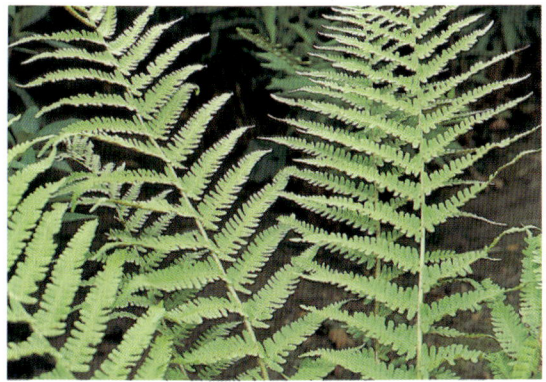

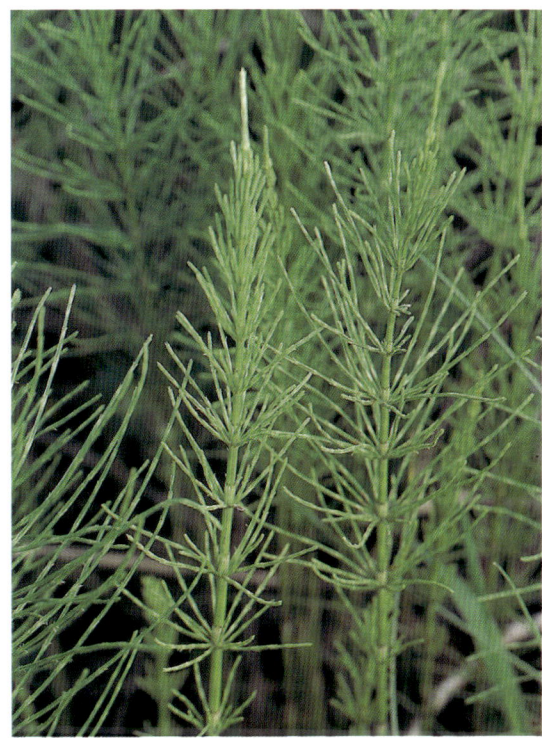

inhale carcinogenic spores when handling the plant. It is known to be addictive and most cases of poisoning occur in late summer and autumn. Bracken also provides a good environment for ticks, which can carry Lyme disease.

The enzyme in bracken (thiaminase) causes thiamine deficiency, which can be treated, if caught early enough, with the daily injection of thiamine (Vitamin B1). If the horse survives, long term rehabilitation incorporating physiotherapy may be required.

Bracken is very difficult to control. If a small quantity is involved it can be regularly cut and removed or uprooted if possible. Large areas and hedges harbouring bracken should be fenced off immediately. Professional help should be sought from agricultural advice agencies to develop a long-term control plan probably using chemicals. Tamworth pigs have been used in trials to uproot bracken in severely infested areas with some success.

HORSETAILS – *Equisetum spp.* (*Equisetaceae*) [also known incorrectly as mare's-tail which is actually *Hippuris vulgaris*, a water plant].

Common horsetail (*see right*) **– *Equisetum arvense*; marsh horsetail – *Equisetum palustre*. There are also about eight other species.**

All species of horsetails look fairly similar, the main differences being variations in stem,

sheath and branching. The stems are jointed and hollow and the branches radiate from the stem. Horsetails can reach 80 cm and grow from a rhizome. They are not flowering plants, but produce spore-bearing cones.

Horsetails contain an alkaloid and also thiaminase – the same enzyme as in bracken. They remain toxic in hay, where they will be readily eaten. Treatment is the same as for bracken poisoning.

Problem areas should be fenced off and professional advice sought to provide a long-term solution.

HEMLOCK – *Conium maculatum* (*Umbelliferae*)
Hemlock is normally biennial but can be annual or perennial. It can reach over 2 m in height, flowers early in the summer and is common on road verges throughout Britain. Although the flowers and leaves are similar to harmless cow parsley (*see page 8, top*), the distinct irregular purple blotches on the stem

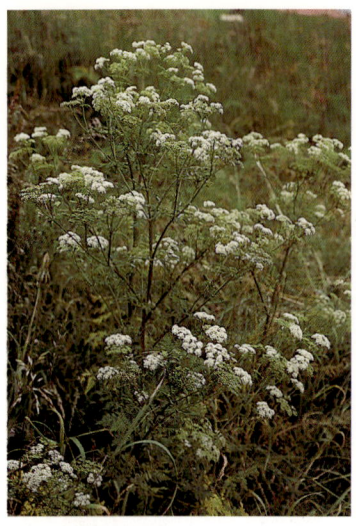 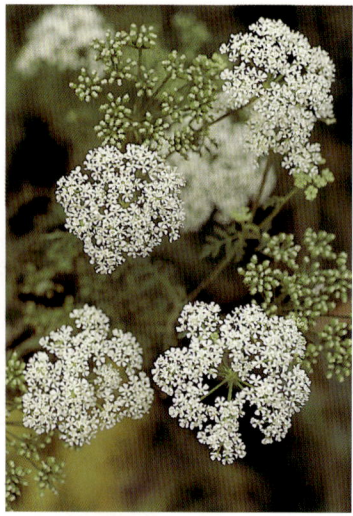 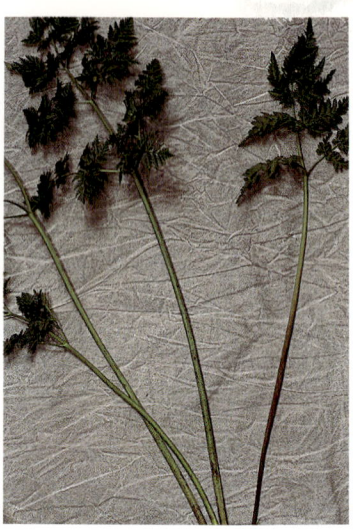

clearly differentiate this plant. The photo *above right* illustrates hemlock leaves (left) compared with cow parsley leaves (right).

The flowers and fruits contain the greatest concentration of the toxic alkaloids. Hemlock is particularly poisonous in dry, hot summers. Although the plant loses a large amount of toxicity when dry, it is best to prevent access to hay containing hemlock. Horses develop signs of severe toxicity after consuming very small quantities. Chances of survival may not be good.

All hemlock plants should be removed and destroyed.

BUTTERCUPS – *Ranunculus spp.* (Ranunculaceae)

Meadow buttercup – *Ranunculus acris* [common buttercup, field buttercup, tall buttercup, crowfoot]

This variety is perennial and is found in pastures and damp areas all over the country although it does not like acid soils.

Bulbous buttercup – *Ranunculus bulbosus* [St Anthony's turnip]
This is also perennial but prefers dry pastures. It is more common in the south.

Celery-leaved crowfoot – *Ranunculus sceleratus* [celery-leaved buttercup, cursed crowfoot]
It is normally annual and is found in muddy areas all over the country.

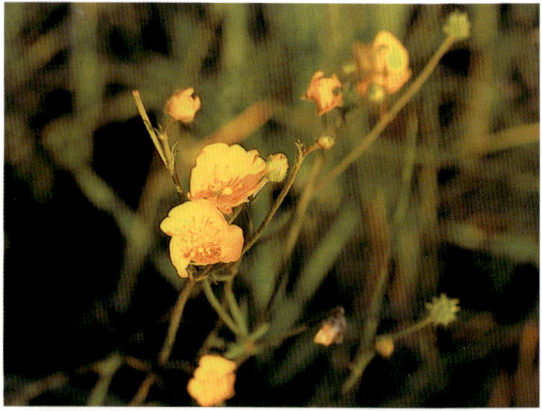

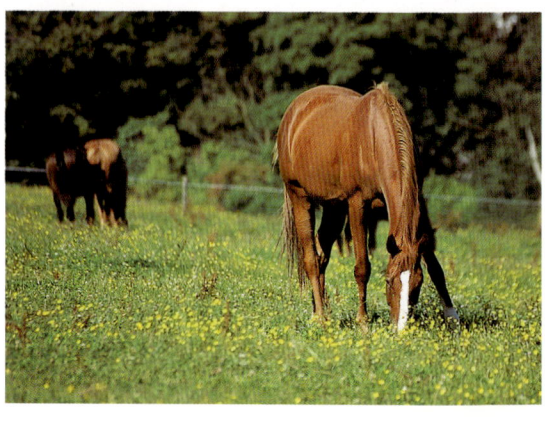

When fresh, all buttercups are poisonous to some extent. In creeping buttercup – *R. repens* – the toxin content is much lower which may explain why it has not been found to be troublesome. The light spots on the leaves distinguish the relatively harmless *R. repens* (left) from the more toxic *R. bulbous* (right) and other buttercups (*see photo below*).

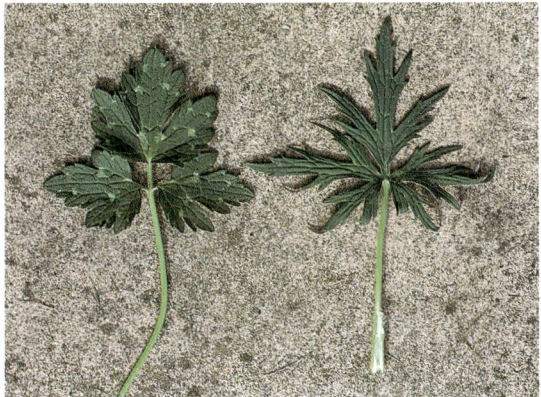

Cattle and sheep are most susceptible so care must be taken when rotating pasture. Buttercups lose their toxicity when dry or in hay.

Horses are unlikely to eat buttercups if on good pasture but are at most risk when on overgrazed or starvation paddocks. It is up to the individual owner to assess the risks. Animals should recover from poisoning in a few days but will be very weak for a while.

Buttercups can be eradicated by 2,4-D weedkiller, although treated areas need to be rested for at least two weeks after spraying since the plants can become more palatable. To deal with a long-term problem, a professional advisor should outline a strategy involving correct drainage and field rotation.

ST JOHN'S WORT – *Hypericum perforatum* (*Clusiaceae*, but can be listed under *Guttiferae*)

Common St John's wort is the plant described here but all of the *Hypericum* species are toxic. It is perennial, reaches 50 cm high and is common in hedgerows and wooded areas throughout Britain. The leaves have tiny

perforations which can be seen when held up to the light, hence the Latin name. Bright yellow flowers with lots of stamens are seen from June to September.

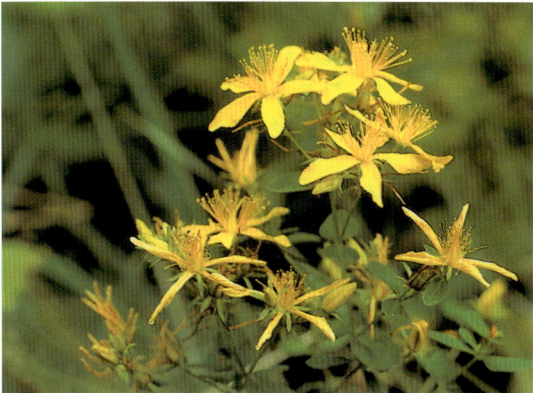

A pigment called hypericine causes photo-sensitisation. This is a condition in which unpigmented skin shown by white markings is easily burned in sunlight and may peel off, leaving painful lesions. When dried, St John's wort is still toxic although to a lesser extent.

Affected animals should be kept in the dark until the toxin has passed through the system and any sunburn should be treated.

Dig out and burn any plants.

THORN APPLE – *Datura stramonium* (*Solanaceae*) [jimsonweed or James Town weed]

This uncommon annual plant can reach a height of 1 m. Trumpet-shaped pinkish flowers

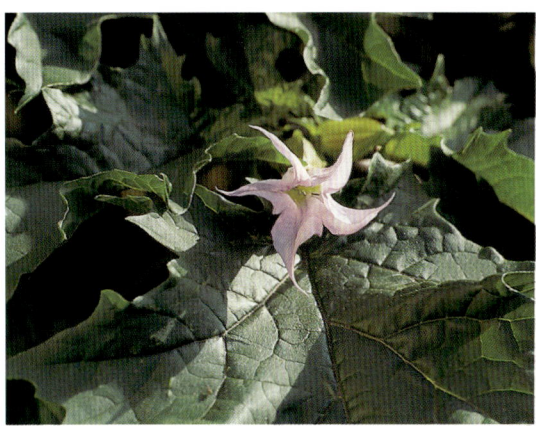

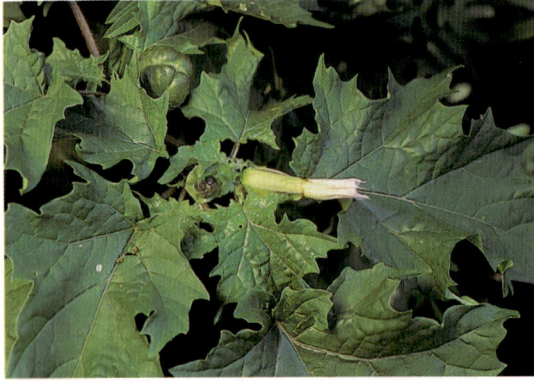

appear from July to August and prickly fruits (*see above*) containing black seeds are formed between August and October. Thorn apple is found on embankments and waste ground in the south of England and in gardens round the country. It contains toxic alkaloids and it remains poisonous when dried and in hay.

Uproot and burn any plants. Wear gloves and take care to keep the plant away from the eyes and face.

LUPIN – *Lupinus x regalis* (*Leguminosae*) [more correctly: Russel lupin]

Lupins are perennial plants which can grow up to 1 m high, are often found in gardens and on roadsides and have compound leaves with radiating leaflets (*see above right*). The flowers, which come in a variety of colours, are seen around May to July, after which the pods are visible. Lupins are still poisonous when dry.

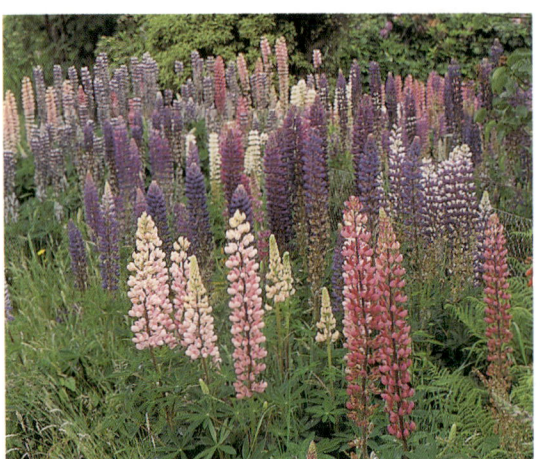

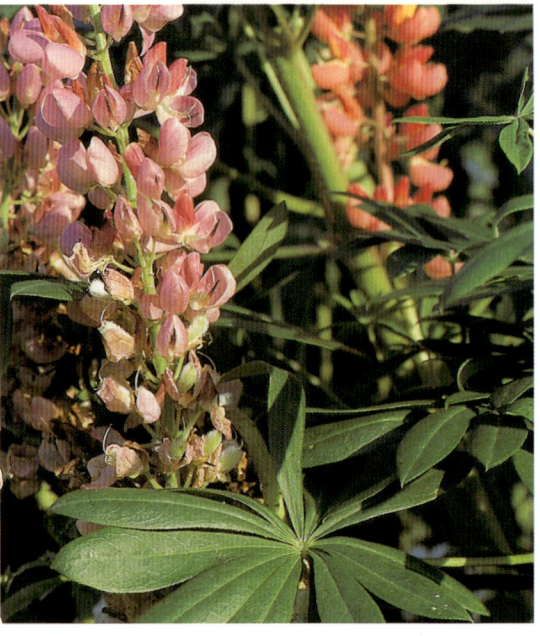

The plant contains both alkaloids, which can cause convulsions, and also substances which can cause reproductive disorders. The mycotoxins produced by fungus found on lupin plants can cause problems.

Lupin plants growing in the field or within reach of the fence should be uprooted and burnt.

WOODLAND PLANTS

FOXGLOVE – *Digitalis purpurea* (*Scrophulariaceae*)

Common throughout Britain, foxgloves are biennial but are occasionally perennial. They can grow up to 1.5 m high. The plant is seen as a rosette of leaves through the first year and into the spring of the second year. The flowers, which appear over the summer, are usually purple or white but can be in pastel colours. In the autumn the plant dries to a stick. *See photos at the top of page 11.*

Toxins are present in foxglove at all stages of growth and when dried. Horses are especially likely to eat it at rosette stage in the

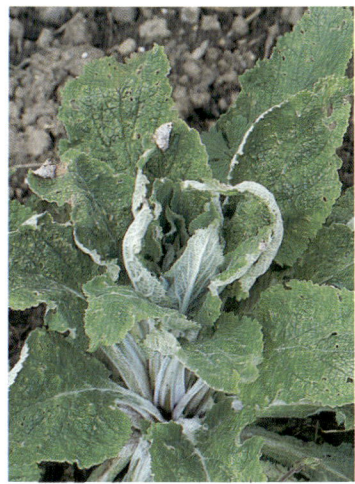 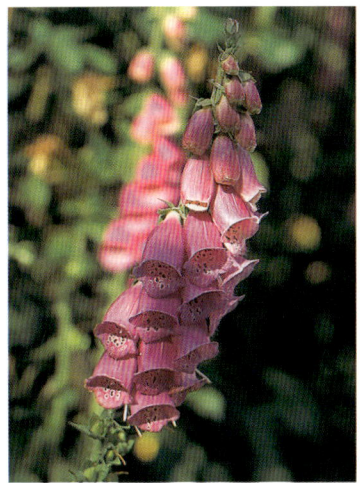 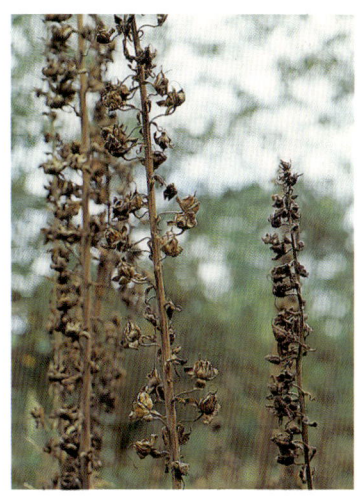

spring when grass is short, or when dried or in hay. Animals can crave it after surviving poisoning.

All plants should be uprooted, taking care to remove plants at rosette stage as well as flowering plants.

CUCKOO PINT – *Arum maculatum* (*Araceae*) [wild arum, lords-and-ladies or wake robin]

Cuckoo pint is a perennial. It is found in shady woody areas and under hedgerows throughout Britain. The pointed leaves are dark green and sometimes have purple blotches. The plant flowers between April and June. Once the leaves have died back

between July and August, red berries appear. *See photos below.*

The poison in cuckoo pint can cause abortion in pregnant mares or can be fatal. Poisoning is rare as usually horses avoid the plant although animals on poor grazing could be tempted.

Plants should be dug up and removed.

RAMSONS – *Allium ursinum* (*Alliaceae*) [wild garlic]

This native bulb is common in damp and wooded areas where its strong onionlike smell clearly indicates its presence. Normally two pointed leaves around 10–20 cm long grow from the bulb. A cluster of tiny white flowers

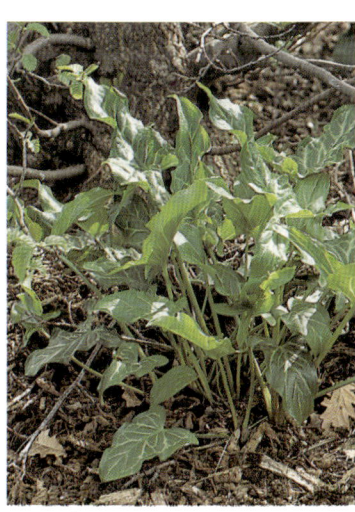 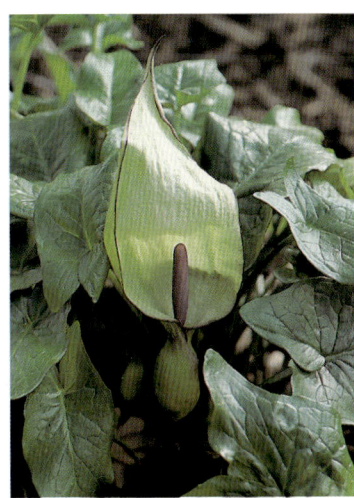 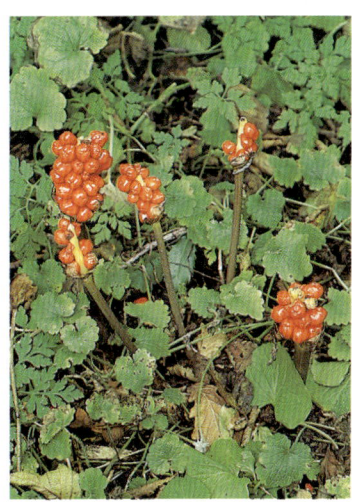

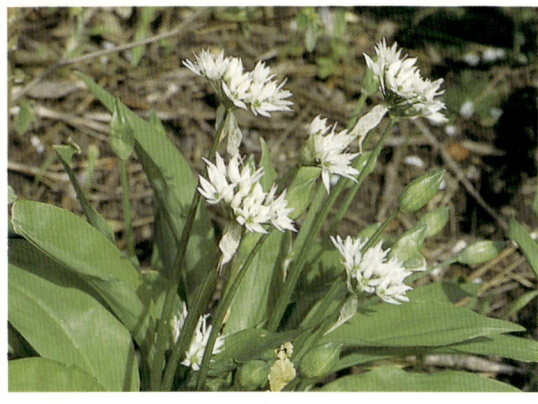

is present on a stalk around April to June (*see above*). The toxin causes, amongst other things, severe anaemia, which could be fatal.

Individual plants can be dug up fairly easily.

MERCURY – *Mercurialis spp.* (*Euphorbiaceae*)

Dog's mercury – *Mercurialis perennis*

Dog's mercury is common in woodland throughout Britain. It grows to 40 cm high from a rhizome and flowers from February to April (*see below*).

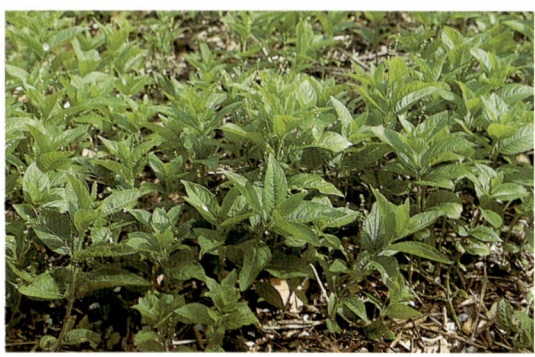

Annual mercury – *Mercurialis annua*

This plant is less common and is found on waste ground and in gardens as a weed and is more common in the south. Annual mercury can grow up to 50 cm tall and the oval leaves are lighter and more shiny than dog's mercury.

The plants are most toxic at flowering and early seeding stages. Poisoning is not common but animals may eat the plant if other food is scarce.

Affected areas should be fenced off or advice taken on methods of removal suitable for the area.

LILY-OF-THE-VALLEY – *Convallaria majalis* (*Liliaceae*)

Lily-of-the-valley is a perennial plant with a creeping rhizome. It is a common garden plant but in nature it prefers woodland areas. It is found throughout Britain and is around 30 cm high. The groups of up to twelve small white flowers (*see below*) can be seen between May and June and the red berries are formed from August to September. There have been few cases of poisoning.

The plant should be uprooted and removed.

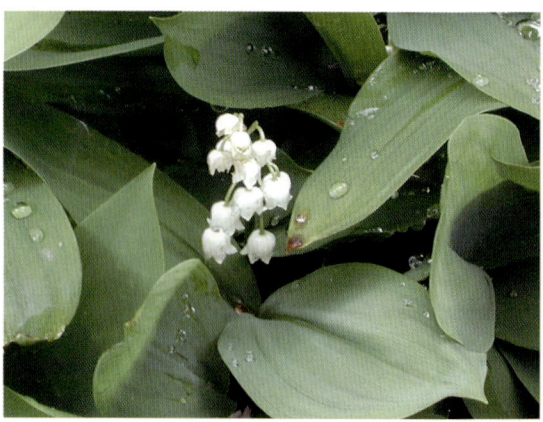

MARSH PLANTS

COWBANE – *Cicuta virosa* (*Umbelliferae*) [water hemlock]

This perennial plant prefers wet areas and ditches and is more common in East Anglia, the Midlands, southern Scotland, and central and northern Ireland. It can reach 130 cm and flowers from July to August (*see page 13, top*). It has a hollow stem and compound leaves and looks similar to the harmless hogweed. They can be differentiated by their

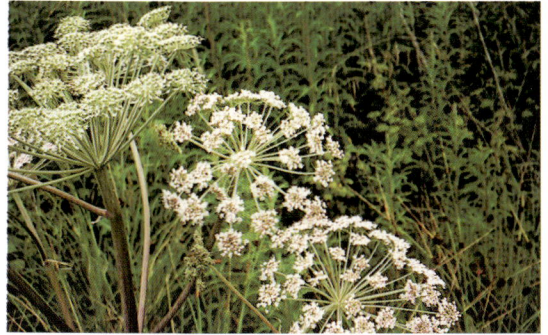

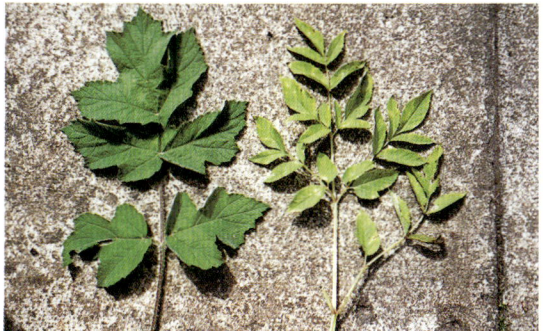

HEMLOCK WATER DROPWORT
Oenanthe crocata (*Umbelliferae*) [dead men's fingers]

Like cowbane, this perennial plant grows in damp places. The toxin it contains is particularly concentrated in winter. The root of the plant is the most poisonous part, therefore there is a great risk from exposed roots when digging ditches for drainage. The plant is still poisonous when dry. The small white flowers appear in May to August. *See photos below.*

Horses are unlikely to survive poisoning.

Take great care when uprooting the plant because it is also highly toxic to humans. The

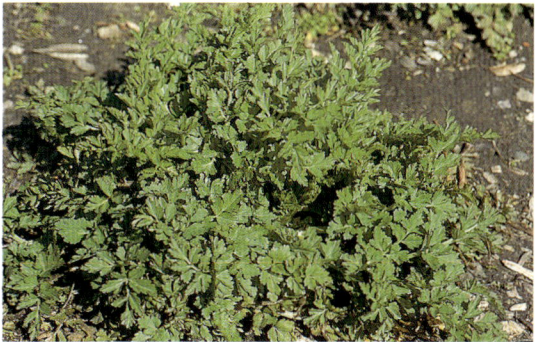

leaves. (*See photo above*: hogweed leaf [left], cowbane leaf [right].)

The toxin is present in the roots and stems. Cowbane is particularly poisonous in late autumn and early winter and is still poisonous when dry.

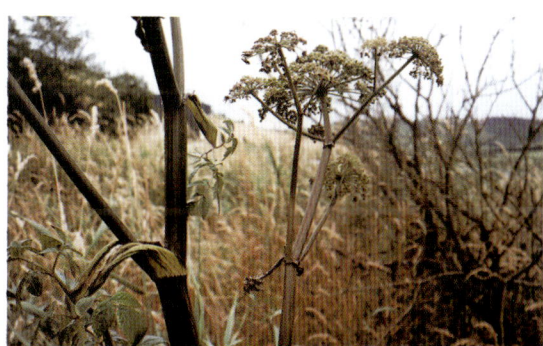

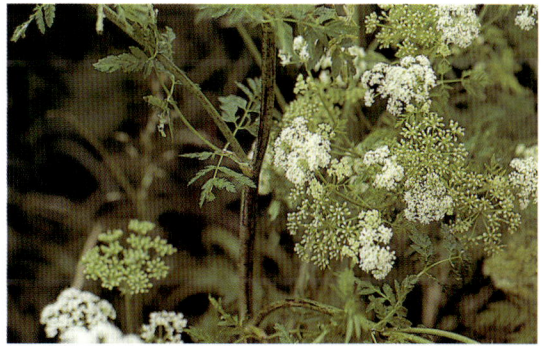

Clinical signs appear within an hour of ingestion. If animals survive up to five to six hours after ingestion of the plant, they generally recover within four to five days.

Cowbane is a nationally scarce plant and is protected by law from being uprooted. The landowner's permission is essential before uprooting plants. If necessary fence off the plants.

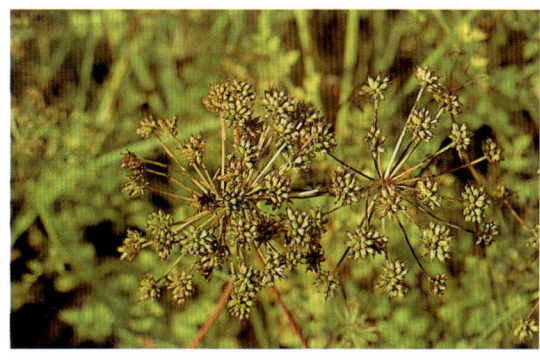

leaves have been mistaken for celery and the tubers for parsnips.

MARSH MARIGOLD – *Caltha palustris* (*Ranunculaceae*)

Marsh marigold is a native perennial and can be found in wet or marshy shady areas all over the country. The bright yellow flowers (*see below*) are seen from March to July. The toxin is the same as that in buttercups.

Remove any plants within reach of horses.

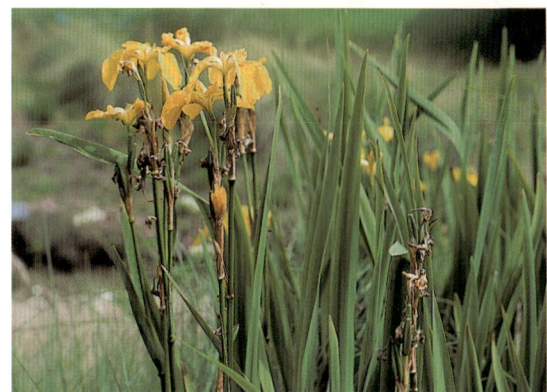

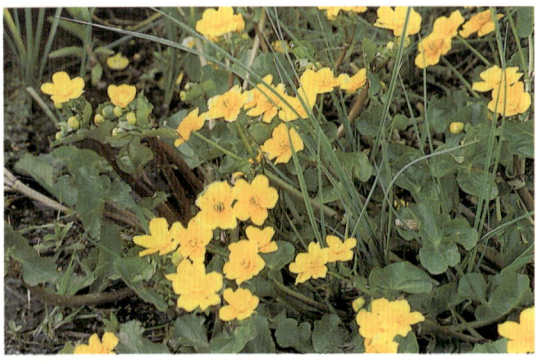

bright yellow flowers can be seen from May to July (*see above*) and around July to August, green capsules form which eventually burst to reveal red berries.

These perennial plants contain a variety of toxins. All parts of the plants are poisonous but particularly the roots. Care must be taken therefore to remove all rhizomes during ditching. Iris are still toxic when dry. Recovery from poisoning is likely within a few days.

Take care to remove all roots when disposing of the plant.

IRIS – *Iris* (*Iridaceae*)

Stinking iris – *Iris foetidissima* [gladdon]

Stinking iris can grow to 70 cm in height and is found in dry places. Purplish flowers are formed between May and July, with bright red berries present from autumn through to spring.

Yellow flag – *Iris pseudacorus*

Yellow flag is taller than stinking iris, reaching up to 1.2 m, and is found in wet areas. The

MONKSHOOD – *Aconitum napellus agg.* (*Ranunculaceae*) [aconite]

This extremely toxic plant is perennial and is normally found in gardens. Where it does occur in the wild it prefers damp, shady areas in the south. It has deeply divided leaves, can reach 1 m in height and the purplish blue flowers are present from May to July after which, seed pods develop. *See photos below.*

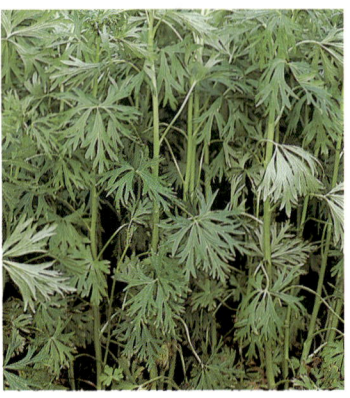

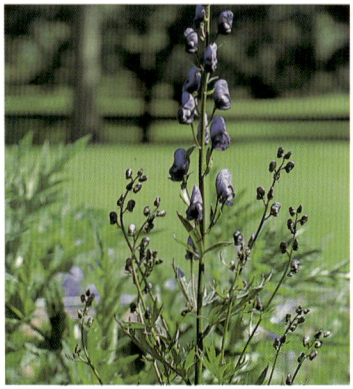

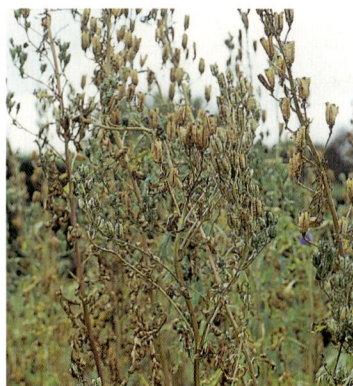

Monkshood contains very poisonous alkaloids and it is estimated that 350 g of dried root would kill a horse.

Plants should be removed and burnt.

MEADOW SAFFRON – *Colchicum autumnale* (*Liliaceae*) [autumn crocus or naked ladies]

Meadow saffron is perennial and is more common in damp areas especially in central England. Long slender leaves grow in spring and die before the pink crocuslike flowers appear in August to October. *See photos below.*

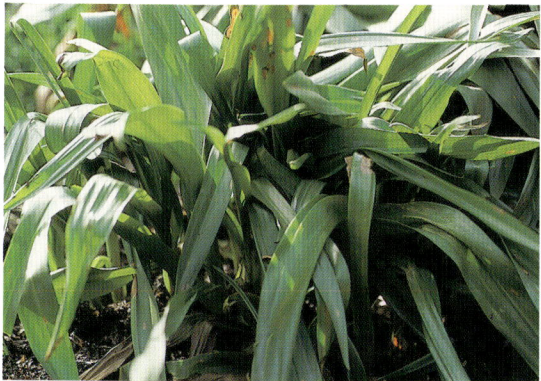

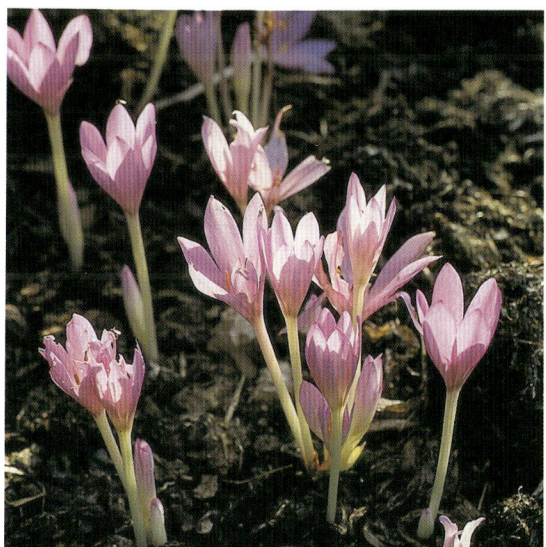

The plant is most toxic during the summer and is still toxic when dry. Signs of poisoning appear after 12–24 hours.

Uproot and burn all plants.

CLIMBING PLANTS

WHITE BRYONY – *Bryonia dioica* (*Cucurbitaceae*) [red bryony]

This is a native perennial climbing plant, climbing by means of tendrils, found on hedges, fences and in woods. It is more common in England and Wales. The stems can grow to around 3 m. Tiny yellowish flowers are produced from May to September and red berries can be seen from August to October. *See photos below.*

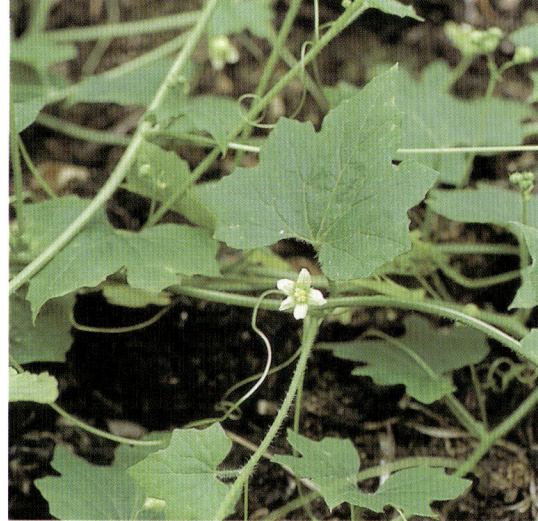

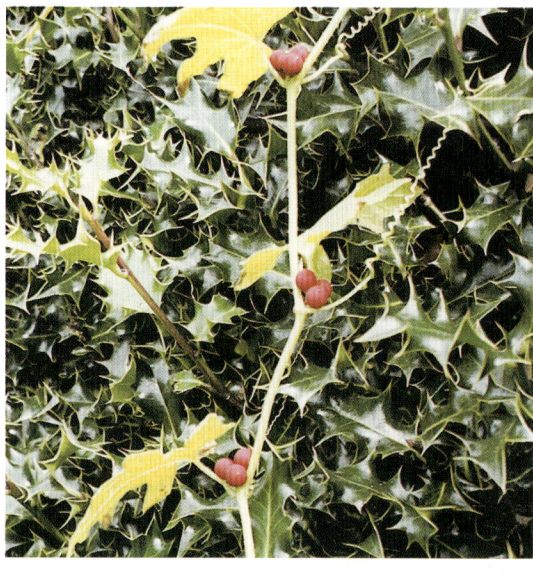

Toxins are present throughout the plant including the roots. The toxicity of the plant decreases with drying.

All plants should be dug up and removed.

WOODY NIGHTSHADE – *Solanum dulcamara* (*Solanaceae*) [bittersweet]

This is a perennial climbing plant which, apart from the woody stems, dies back in winter. It is found throughout Britain on trees and hedges or growing along the ground. There are two different leaf shapes, either oval or heart shaped, which can have up to four lobes near the base of the leaf. Purple flowers with yellow centres appear in the summer. Green berries appear between September and October and eventually ripen to red. *See below.*

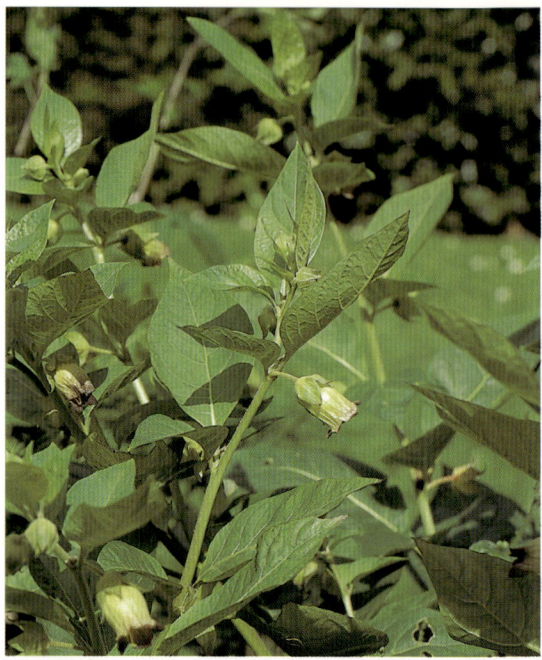

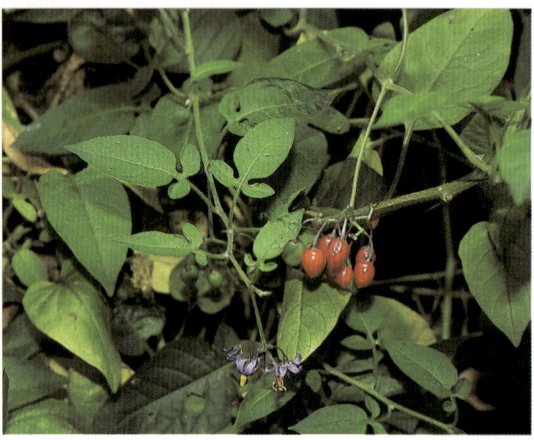

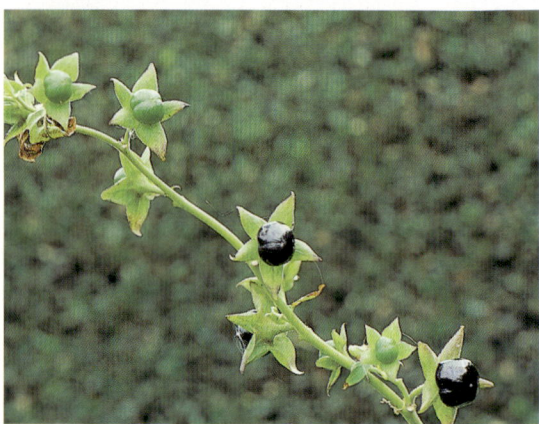

Fortunately poisoning is rare.

Remove all branches climbing over hedges and walls, as well as the root.

DEADLY NIGHTSHADE – *Atropa belladonna* (*Solanaceae*) [dwale or belladonna]

A perennial plant with purple flowers appearing from June to August. Green berries ripen to black in the autumn and resemble huge blackcurrants. *See photos right.*

All parts of the plant are extremely poisonous. Fortunately the plant is rarely eaten.

Uproot and burn all plants.

TREES AND SHRUBS

LABURNUM – *Laburnum anagyroides* (*Leguminosae*) [golden chain or golden rain]

Laburnum is a tree that can grow to around 7m high. From May to June bright yellow pendant sprays up to 20 cm long appear, after which green pods are formed. The pods dry and then burst open to reveal small black seeds. The open pods can stay on the plant over the winter. *See photos on page 17, top.*

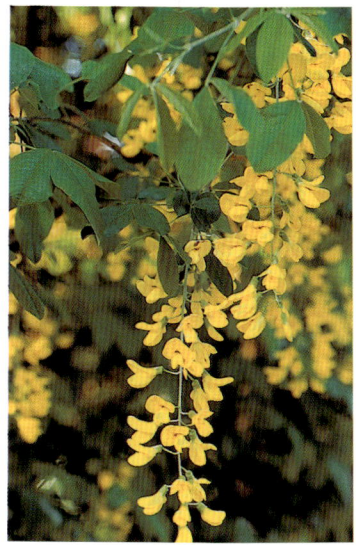
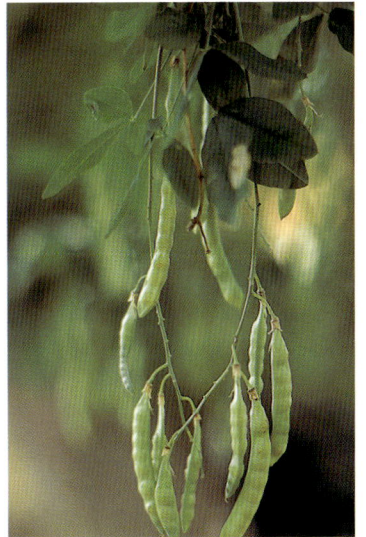
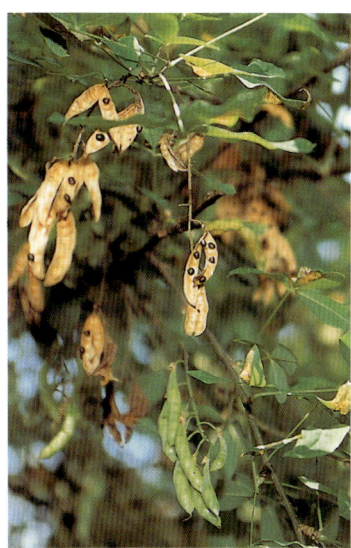

The toxin in laburnum varies in quantity from plant to plant. All parts of the tree are toxic but the bark and seeds are especially poisonous. The leaves become less toxic and the flowers and fruits more so as they develop. Poisoning can result in death.

Trees should be fenced off and the ground should be checked for fallen leaves or seedpods. Alternatively laburnum trees could be cut down. If laburnum is growing as part of a hedge it could be cut out and replaced by a non-toxic plant.

YEW – *Taxus spp. (Taxaceae)*

English yew, common yew, yew – *Taxus baccata*
The tiny yellow flowers can be seen from March to April with male and female flowers on different trees. Attractive bright red berries appear around August to September. *See photos right.*

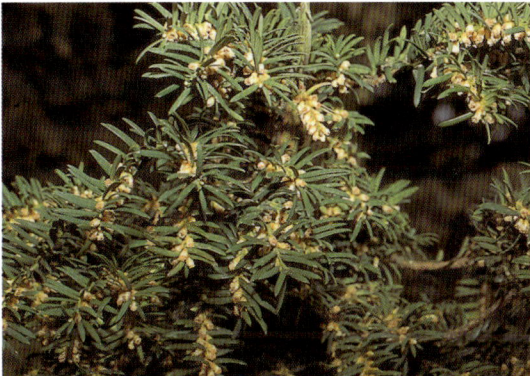

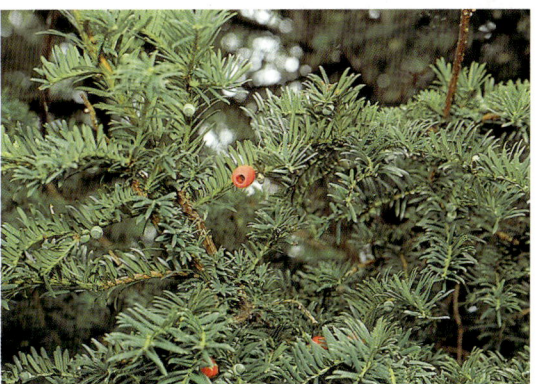

TOXIC TETHERING POSTS

Always check that horses are not tied to poisonous trees.

Irish yew, churchyard yew – *Taxus baccata var fastigiata*
The branches of this species are more upright, in contrast to the almost horizontal branches of the English yew.

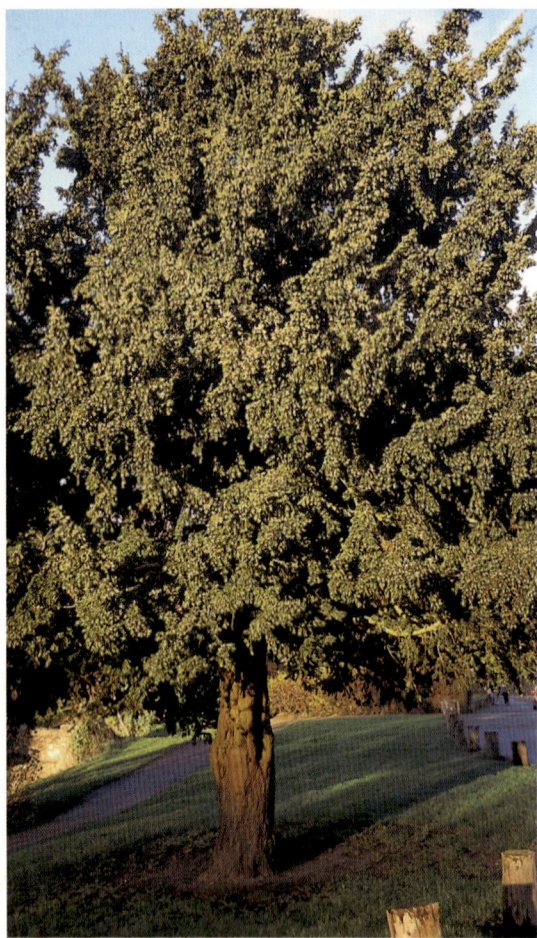

OAK AND ACORNS – *Quercus spp.* (*Fagaceae*)

Pedunculate oak or English oak – *Quercus robur*

This native tree is common in England and the south of Scotland. It can be around 30 m high and the leaves have very short stalks. The acorns, which develop in the autumn, do have stalks.

Sessile oak or durmast oak – *Quercus petraea*

This species is seen more often in north and west Britain. The acorns have no stalks or very short stalks up to 1 cm long.

Oaks are mostly deciduous trees with distinctive deeply lobed leaves. Flowers appear around April to May and acorns are produced in September and October. *See below.*

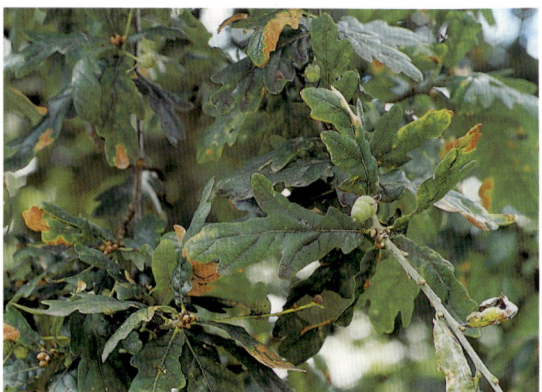

Yews are evergreen trees found in hedges, gardens and churchyards throughout the country and may be the most poisonous tree in Europe. *See above.* Yew is most toxic in winter, when animals are more likely to eat it.

The fatal dose is thought to be 0.5–2 g per kg of body weight. Normally the animal is found dead since death is rapid. If the animal is still alive when discovered, the stomach contents need to be removed.

The tree should be removed if practicable and if it is not protected, or should be securely fenced off. Horses can escape and eat yew in winter when desperate for green food. Ensure horses have no access to hedge cuttings containing yew.

Take no risks with yew.

There is conflicting evidence on poisoning and therefore is it difficult to assess how much of a risk there is from oak. However it is better to be safe and prevent horses having access to these trees. Tannins are the main poisonous substances found in all parts of the tree with more in young leaves and green acorns. The tannin content of the sap is at its highest in the spring.

Oak and acorns can be so addictive that animals that have only just managed to survive poisoning may actively seek out oak again. Reports of poisoning are more common in the autumn when acorns are more abundant. Feeding bran and hay may reduce the severe effects of poisoning.

Oak trees must be fenced off. Horses which have suffered from oak poisoning may break down fences to get to oak trees. Pick up acorns that fall onto the pasture.

BOX – *Buxus sempervirens* (*Buxaceae*)

Box is an evergreen tree or shrub with grey bark and fragrant foliage. The flowers which appear between March and May are yellow and very small. Black seeds contained within dry capsules appear in the late summer. Box can be found in hedges, woods and scrubland. *See right.*

All parts of the plant contain poisonous steroidal alkaloids. It has been estimated that only 750 g of this plant would be enough to kill a horse.

Hedges containing box must be fenced off. Ensure that horses have no access to hedge cuttings.

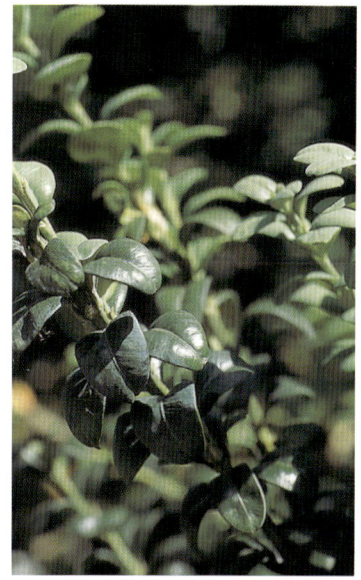

CHERRY LAUREL – *Prunus laurocerasus* (*Rosaceae*)

Cherry laurel is an introduced evergreen shrub, which can reach heights of 5–6 m or can be found growing as part of a hedge. The thick shiny green leaves are around 15 cm long, smelling of almonds when crushed. White flowers develop in the spring and fruits ripen from green to black in late summer. *See photos below.*

The cynanogenic glycosides in the plant lead to cyanide poisoning. Affected animals

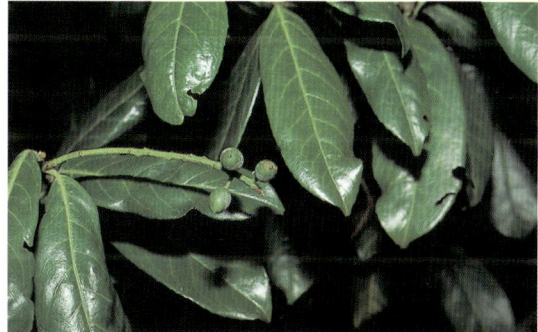

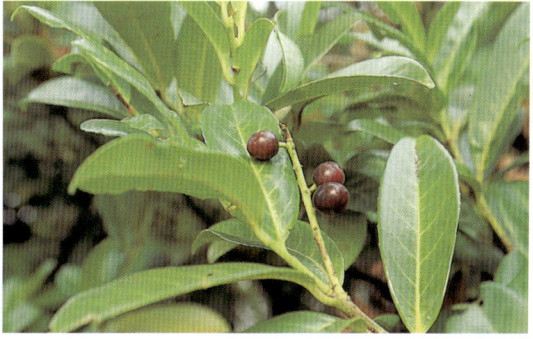

are likely to be found dead, but if still alive the stomach contents will need to be emptied.

Shrubs and hedges must be fenced off and any overhanging branches cut back. Take care that horses have no access to hedge cuttings.

PRIVET – *Ligustrum spp.* (*Oleaceae*)

Wild privet – *Ligustrum vulgare*

This deciduous shrub is found throughout the country. From June to July white flowers can be seen. Green berries ripen to black around September to October.

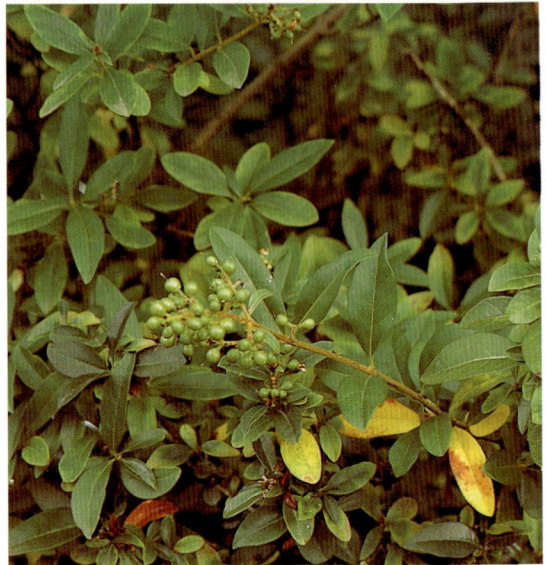

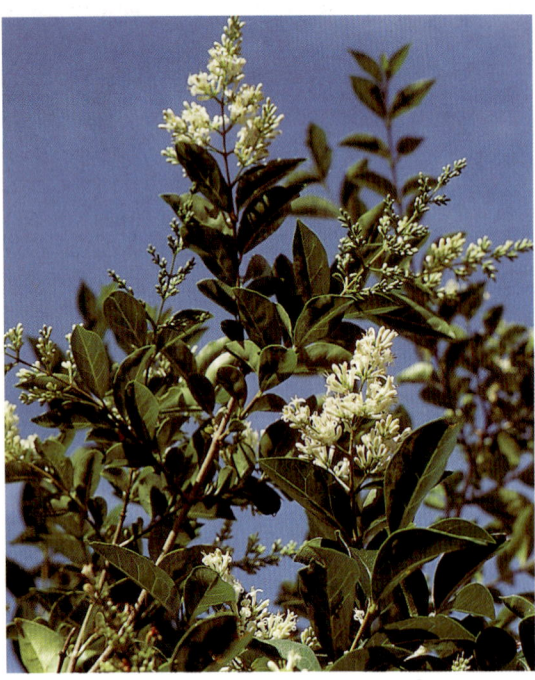

Garden privet – *Ligustrum ovalifolium*

This introduced species of privet can be evergreen. Like common privet it is found all over Britain, but the leaves of this variety are more oval and the flowers are longer.

Both types of privet are found in hedges and gardens. The toxic glycoside is present in all parts of the plant and the berries are particularly poisonous. Privet poisoning can cause death within four to forty-eight hours.

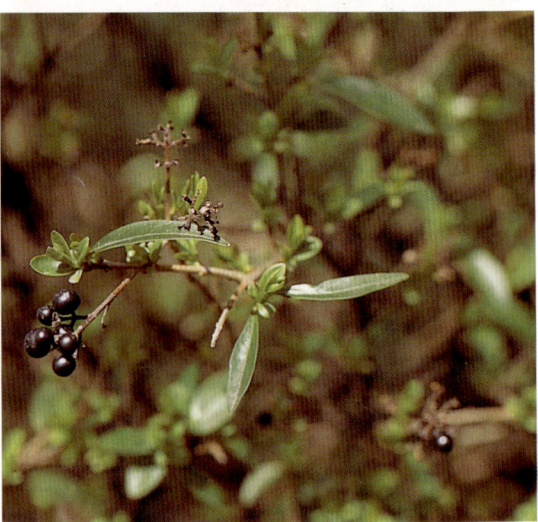

Fence off privet hedges and prevent access to hedge clippings.

No chances should be taken with privet.

RHODODENDRON – *Rhododendron ponticum* (*Ericaceae*) [common rhododendron or pontic rhododendron]

Rhododendron is a branched evergreen shrub reaching 3 m. It is often found in woods, gardens, parks and hedges across the country. The purple flowers are formed in the spring, and there are different colours in other cultivated species.

The leaves and flowers contain toxins which can cause death. Treatment involves the removal of the stomach contents.

All rhododendron bushes and hedges must be fenced off and care taken with hedge clippings.

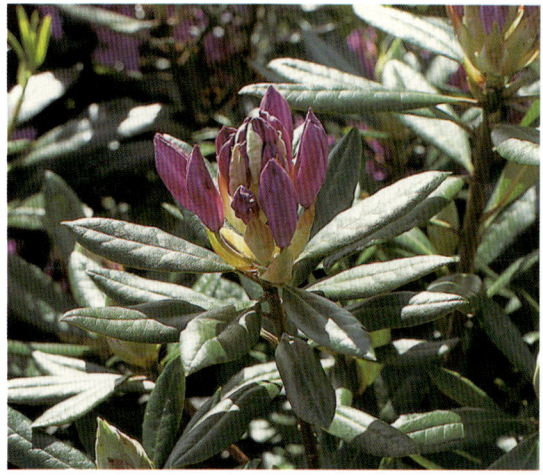

> ### DECIDUOUS COUSIN
>
> Azaleas, which are deciduous rhododendrons, are also poisonous.

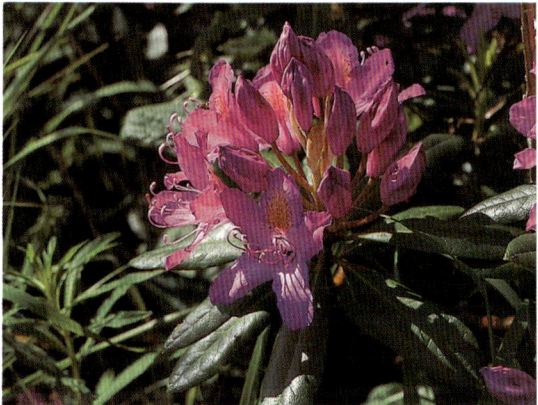

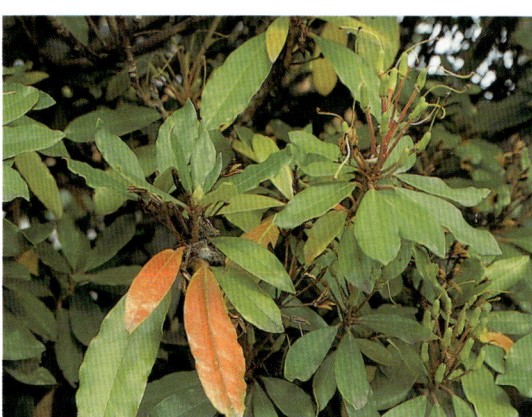

POTENTIALLY DANGEROUS PLANTS

The plants listed in this section come under one of the following categories:
- plants that are very poisonous but horses would rarely come across them;
- plants that horses rarely eat even when in abundance;
- plants that are potentially poisonous if eaten in large quantities.

Details of where photographs of these plants can be found are given on page 23.

ALDER BUCKTHORN – *Frangula alnus (Rhamnaceae)* Can cause colic and diarrhoea. Take care with hedge clippings.

BEECH – *Fagus sylvatica (Fagaceae)* Can be found in hedges or as a large tree. The beech nuts present the main danger, so remove all nuts which have fallen onto the pasture.

BINDWEED – *Convolvulus arvensis (Convolvulaceae)* Potential danger if animals are hungry.

BLACK BRYONY – *Tamus communis (Dioscoreaceae)* Can be seen climbing trees and hedges.

BLACK NIGHTSHADE/ GARDEN NIGHTSHADE – *Solanum nigram (Solanaceae)* Conflicting accounts of danger as toxin levels vary from plant to plant. Some varieties are developing resistance to herbicides.

BROOM – *Cytisus scoparius (Leguminosae)* A shrub found mostly on waste land and in gardens. A very large dose could cause poisoning.

BUCKTHORN – *Rhamnus cathartica (Rhamnaceae)*
See alder buckthorn.

CASTOR OIL PLANT* – *Ricinus communis
(Euphorbiaceae)* Very toxic but poisoning is rare.

CHARLOCK – *Sinapsis arvensis (Cruciferae)* Weed
found on arable ground. The seeds are poisonous.

CHICKWEED – *Stellaria media (Caryophyllaceae)* Can
cause poisoning

CLOVER – *Trifolium spp (Leguminosae)* Too much clover
on pasture can cause a range of problems.

COLUMBINE – *Aquilegia vulgaris (Ranunculaceae)*
Potentially poisonous.

CORNCOCKLE – *Agrostemma githago
(Caryophyllaceae)* Have not been many cases recently
as the plant is fairly rare.

DELPHINIUM/LARKSPUR – *Delphinium spp. Consolida
ajacis (Ranunculaceae)* Normally found in gardens, but
also in the wild. Could cause fatal poisoning. Beware of
garden waste.

FOOL'S PARSLEY – *Aethusa cynapium (Umbelliferae)*
Poisoning is possible but the plant is safe in hay.

GREATER CELANDINE – *Chelidonium majus
(Papaveraceae)* Has orange sap. Rarely causes
problems.

GREATER SPEARWORT – *Ranunculus lingua
(Ranunculaceae)* May cause symptoms similar to
buttercup poisoning.

GROUND IVY – *Glechoma hederacea (Labiatae)* Horses
are unlikely to eat it.

HELLEBORE – *Hellebores spp. (Ranunculaceae)* More
commonly found in gardens.

HEMP NETTLE – *Galeopsis ladanum (Labiatae)* No
recent cases of poisoning.

HENBANE – *Hyoscyamus niger (Solanaceae)* Extremely
toxic but no recent cases of poisoning.

HERB PARIS – *Paris quadrifolia (Liliaceae)* Tastes
unpleasant therefore poisoning is unlikely. Can be a
protected species in some areas.

HOLLY – *Ilex aquifolium (Aquifoliaceae)* Can cause
poisoning when eaten because no other food available.

HORSE RADISH – *Armoracia rusticana (Cruciferae)*
Unpleasant taste but can cause fatal poisoning.

IVY – *Hedera helix (Araliaceae)* If large quantities are
consumed this will cause illness.

LESSER SPEARWORT – *Ranunculus flammula
(Ranunculaceae)* As for greater spearwort.

LINSEED/FLAX* – *Linum usitatissimum (Linaceae)*
The danger occurs if the seed has not been cooked
properly before being fed to horses.

MELILOT – *Melilotus spp. (Leguminosae)* Only a
problem if dried in hay which, fortunately, is unlikely.

**MEZEREON/SPURGE OLIVE/FLAX/DWARF
BAY/WILD PEPPER** – *Daphne mezereum
(Thymelaeaceae)* More common in gardens. Should
not be given as a worm treatment as it causes
poisoning and colic and can be fatal. This is a scarce
plant nationally. *See below.*

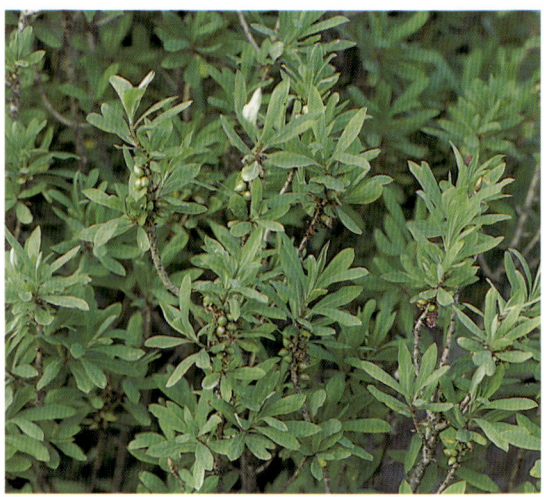

MILK VETCHES – *Astragalus spp. (Leguminosae)* Have
not caused many problems in Britain.

POPPY (OPIUM) – *Papaver somniferum (Papaveraceae)*
Unlikely to cause problems.

POTATO* – *Solanum tuberosum (Solanaceae)* Horses
should not be fed potatoes or any part of the plant. *See
page 23, top left.*

RAPE/COLE/COLZA – *Brassica napus (Cruciferae)*
Best avoided. It is thought that it could cause
respiratory problems from airborne pollen.

**SCARLET PIMPERNEL/SHEPHERD'S
WEATHERGLASS** – *Anagallis arvensis (Primulaceae)*
Conflicting accounts of poisoning – possibly different
effects on different animals.

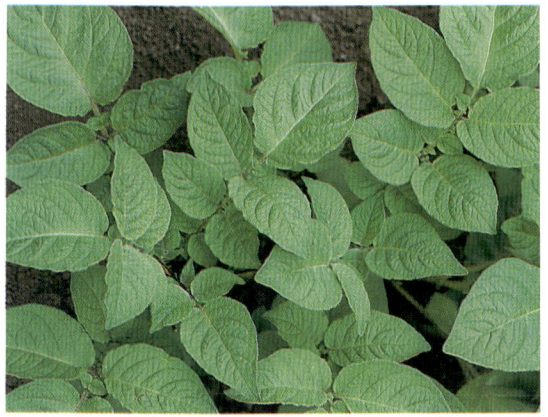

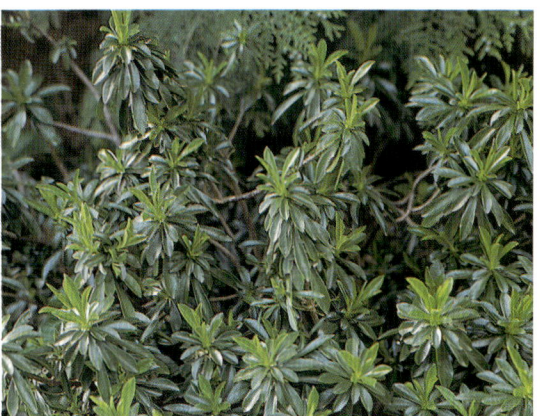

SORREL – *Rumex spp. (Polygonaceae)* Has reportedly caused poisoning in horses.

SPURGES * – *Euphorbia spp. (Euphorbiaceae)* Potentially dangerous but there have been no reports in this country.

SPURGE LAUREL/WOOD LAUREL/COPSE LAUREL – *Daphne laureola (Thymelaeaceae)* Can cause fatal poisoning in horses. *See right, above.*

WOOD ANEMONE – *Anemone nemorosa (Ranunculaceae)* Has not caused many cases of poisoning, but could cause similar symptoms to buttercup poisoning. *See right.*

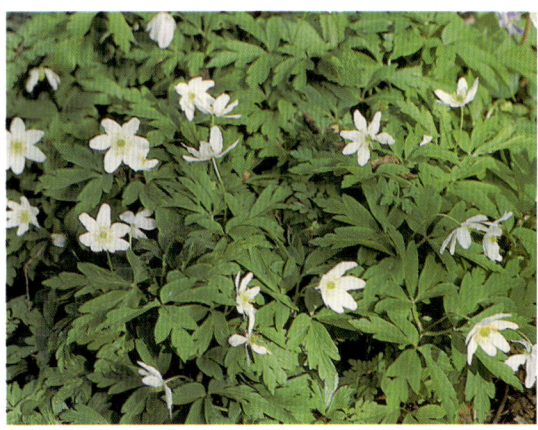

Photographs of most of these plants can be found in *Wild Flowers of Britain*, by Roger Phillips, published by Macmillan Reference, 1994, ISBN 0 330 25183X.

Photographs of those plants marked * are in *Poisonous Plants and Fungi in Britain – Animal and Human Poisoning*, by Marion Cooper and Anthony Johnson, published by The Stationery Office 1998, ISBN 0 112 429815.

FURTHER INFORMATION

Barrier Animal Health Care (Barrier H™ herbicide)
36 & 37 Haverscroft Industrial Estate,
New Road,
Attleborough, Norfolk, NR17 1YE
Tel: 01953 456 363
www.ragwort.com

Veterinary Poisons Information Unit,
National Poisons Information Service,
Leeds General Infirmary,
Great George Street,
Leeds, LS1 3EX
Tel: 01132 430715

British Horse Society Welfare Department,
Stoneleigh Deer Park,
Kenilworth,
Warwickshire, CV8 2XZ
Tel: 01926 707700

Equine Behaviour Forum,
63 Chaigley Road,
Longridge,
Lancashire, PR3 3TQ
http://www.gla.ac.uk/External/EBF/

ACKNOWLEDGEMENTS

I would like to thank Angela Kilday of the Royal Botanic Garden Edinburgh for arranging permission for me to photograph plants in the garden. My special thanks go to Mr D. R. McLean of the Royal Botanic Garden Edinburgh for his invaluable technical assistance and also to Derek Braid for his considerable effort photographing plants over many months.

For the photograph of the ragwort rosette on page 5, my thanks to Barrier Animal Health Care, 36 & 37 Haverscroft Industrial Estate, New Road, Attleborough, Norfolk, NR17 1YE. Tel: 01953 456 363, and for the photograph of the 'Ecopuller' on page 6 my thanks to Alvan Blanch, Chelworth, Malmesbury, Wiltshire, SN16 9SG   Tel: 01666 577 333

British Library Cataloguing-in-Publication Data.
A catalogue record for this book is available from the British Library

ISBN 0.85131.804.5

Published in Great Britain in 2001 by
J. A. Allen an imprint of Robert Hale Ltd.,
Clerkenwell House, 45–47 Clerkenwell Green,
London EC1R 0HT

Design and Typesetting by Paul Saunders
Series editor Jane Lake
Colour processing by Tenon & Polert Colour Processing Ltd., Hong Kong
Printed in Malta by Gutenberg Press Ltd.